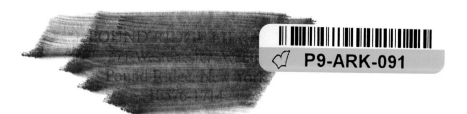

Girls' Health™

Menstruation

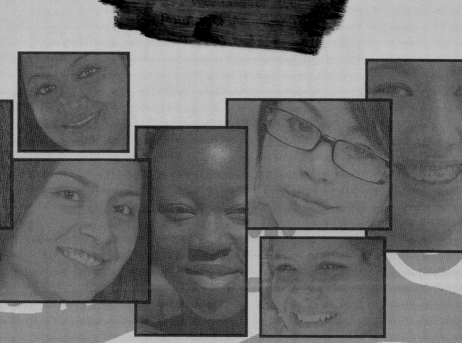

Ann Byers

rosen publishing's
rosen central®

New York

Published in 2008 by The Rosen Publishing Group, Inc.
29 East 21st Street, New York, NY 10010

First Edition

Library of Congress Cataloging-in-Publication Data

Byers, Ann.
Menstruation / Ann Byers.—1st ed.
    p. cm.—(Girls' health)
Includes bibliographical references and index.
ISBN-13: 978-1-4042-0965-7
ISBN-10: 1-4042-0965-4
1. Menstruation--Juvenile literature.
I. Title.
QP263.B944 2007
612.6'62—dc22

                                                    2007001034

Manufactured in the United States of America

Contents

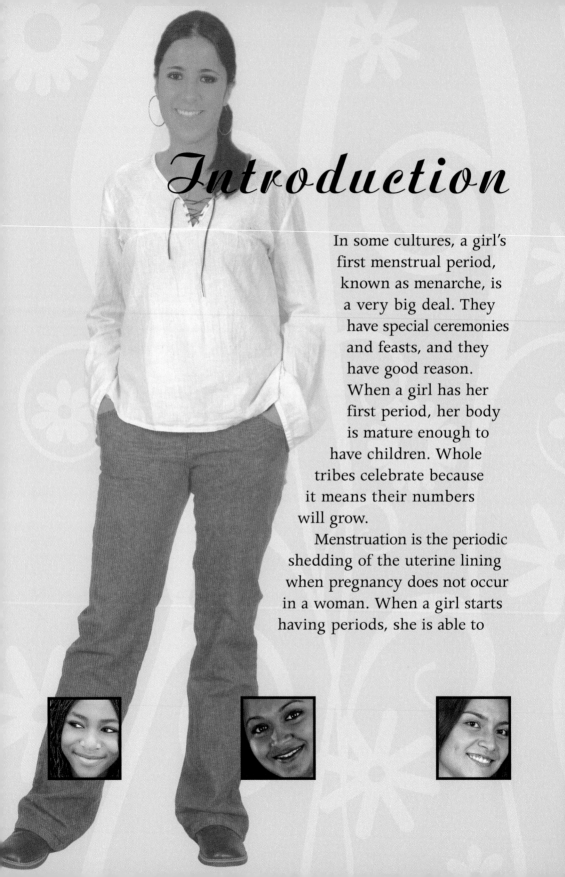

Introduction

In some cultures, a girl's first menstrual period, known as menarche, is a very big deal. They have special ceremonies and feasts, and they have good reason. When a girl has her first period, her body is mature enough to have children. Whole tribes celebrate because it means their numbers will grow.

Menstruation is the periodic shedding of the uterine lining when pregnancy does not occur in a woman. When a girl starts having periods, she is able to

get pregnant. When she reaches menopause—the cessation of the menstrual cycle usually occurring around age fifty—she cannot get pregnant anymore.

When a female baby is born, she already has all the equipment she needs to have a baby. She has a uterus, two fallopian tubes, and two ovaries. These are the organs of her reproductive system. They enable her to produce another human being.

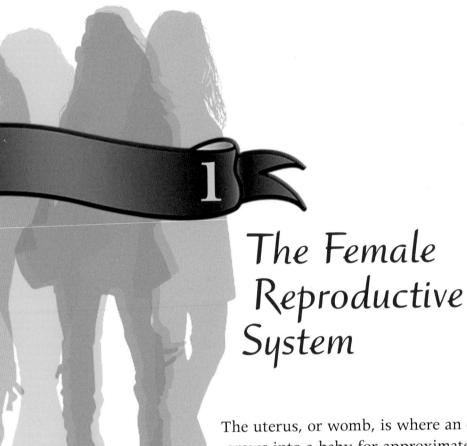

The Female Reproductive System

The uterus, or womb, is where an egg grows into a baby for approximately nine months before it is born. The uterus, located in the lower abdomen, is shaped like an upside-down pear, with the narrow end joined to the top of the vagina. The uterus is hollow and made of muscles that are some of the strongest in the body. They have to be strong to push a baby out. The organ is small—not quite as big as a fist, and about 1 inch (2.5 centimeters) thick. It weighs only 1 to 1.5 ounces (30–40 grams). It can grow large enough to hold a baby that is 9 pounds (4 kilograms) or bigger.

On each side of the uterus is a fallopian tube. These two tubes are attached to the uterus on one end and open on the other. They are thin tubes, like tiny straws, each about 4 inches (10 cm) long. The eggs travel in these tubes to the uterus. Very fine hairs inside the tubes move the eggs along.

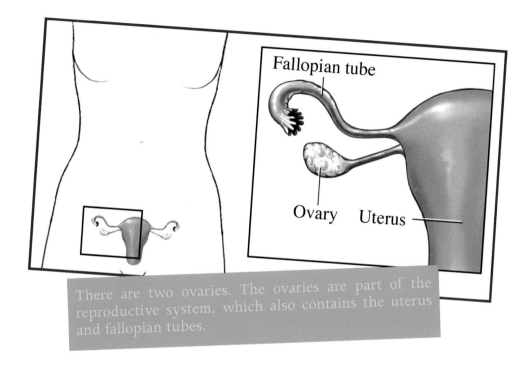

There are two ovaries. The ovaries are part of the reproductive system, which also contains the uterus and fallopian tubes.

The eggs begin in the ovaries. Girls have two ovaries, one on each side of the uterus next to the open ends of the fallopian tubes. They are shaped like, and are about the same size of, almonds. When a baby girl is born, her ovaries already have all the eggs she will need to have children. In fact, she has more than she will ever need—about 1,000,000 to 2,000,000. These are not mature eggs. They do not even begin to mature until she is at least eight years old, and more often ten or twelve years of age or even older as she enters puberty.

When the first egg matures, a girl's reproductive system goes into operation. The egg moves from the ovary in which it was formed into the fallopian tube next to that ovary. From there, it

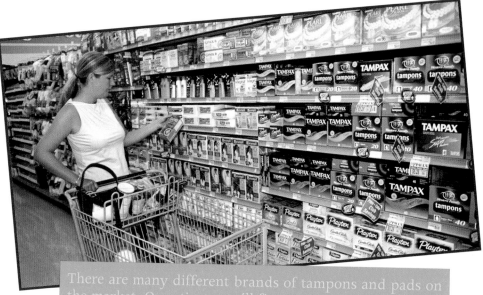

There are many different brands of tampons and pads on the market. Over time, you'll figure out which one is best for you.

travels to the uterus. During the time the egg is developing and moving, the uterus is getting ready to receive it. The body sends blood to the tissues that line the walls of the uterus. The lining is called the endometrium. The endometrium grows new layers so it becomes thick and soft. This makes the uterus a safe place for the growing baby. It also supplies the nutrients the baby needs to grow. Fertilization occurs when a sperm from a male joins with the female's egg while it is traveling in the fallopian tube. It will then attach itself to the cushiony lining of the uterus.

If the egg is not fertilized, the uterus does not need the extra blood and added layers, so it gets rid of them. Along with the egg that has decomposed, blood and some of the tissue that makes up the endometrium flow out through the cervix, the

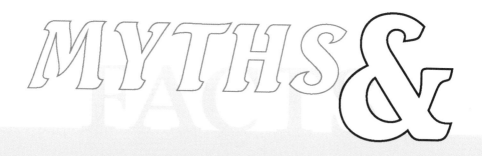

MYTH Your period can be so heavy, you can bleed to death.

FACT Most of the discharge is endometrial tissue, not blood. The normal amount of blood lost during a period is 1 to 2 ounces (30 to 60 ml).

MYTH You can't get pregnant if you have sex during your period.

FACT You are not likely to get pregnant during your period, but you can get pregnant anytime you have sex. Sperm can live for three to five days, and if your cycle is very short, you can ovulate almost right after your period ends.

MYTH Tampons can get lost inside the body.

FACT Your vagina is only about 5 inches (13 cm) long. The opening at the top of the vagina that leads to the uterus is very small, much too small for a tampon to go in.

MYTH Virgins cannot use tampons.

FACT Virgins can use tampons, and using tampons doesn't change you from being a virgin.

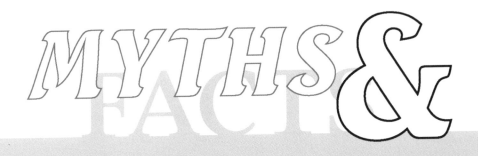

MYTH Tampons cause cancer.

FACT Tampons do not cause cancer. They might, in rare cases, contribute to toxic shock syndrome, an infection that can be cured.

MYTH Menstruating makes you weak, so you need to rest during your period.

FACT You do not lose enough blood to become weak, and exercising keeps you healthy.

opening at the bottom of the uterus, through the vagina, and out the woman's body. This is menstruation. Although most people call menstruation "bleeding," the discharge—what comes out—is only partly blood. Most of it is the extra uterine lining. The flow lasts just a week, or even less. Sanitary pads or tampons are used during menstruation to absorb this flow.

If a fertilized egg plants itself in the uterus, this is the beginning of pregnancy. Menstruation stops until after a baby is born or the uterus is emptied. When no fertilized egg is in the uterus, the process repeats itself about once a month. The word "menstruation" comes from the Latin word for "month." Because the shedding happens regularly, we call it the menstrual cycle. When it happens, we say a girl has her period because the

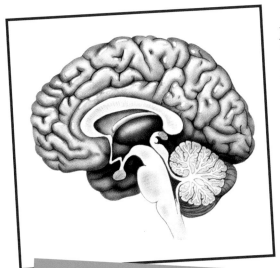

In the image above, the hypothalamus is the purple area. Just below it, in yellow, is the pituitary gland. Both regulate many of the body's functions, including menstruation.

process happens periodically. What makes it happen? What makes an egg mature and start the process? How does the uterus know when to prepare?

Hormones

Hormones are chemicals that control how different parts of the body operate. The body makes more than forty kinds of hormones, each with a specific message for a specific organ. The organs of the female reproductive system are controlled by a chain of hormones that begins in the brain.

In the center of the brain are the hypothalamus (the command center for the entire body) and the pituitary gland (the master gland). They regulate growth, hunger, sleep, and many other activities, including reproduction. First, the hypothalamus sends a hormone to the pituitary gland. Then the pituitary gland sends hormones to the ovaries. Each egg is inside a pocket, or sac, called a follicle. When the ovaries get the message, several eggs start to develop. As the eggs mature, the ovaries release the hormone estrogen. This hormone is what makes the lining of the uterus, the endometrium, thicken. When the uterus is ready for an egg, the hypothalamus sends another hormone to the pituitary gland that starts the process of getting an egg to the waiting uterus. The pituitary gland sends a new type of hormone to the ovaries that makes the most mature follicle burst open and release its egg. The egg leaves the ovary, finds its way into a fallopian tube, and from there travels to the uterus.

Now the broken follicle begins to produce two important hormones: estrogen and progesterone. They are often called female hormones. An egg cannot grow properly without a good supply of these two hormones. The follicle produces these hormones the whole time the egg is in the uterus. But if the egg is not fertilized, it dies and the follicle stops making hormones. Without the hormones, the blood supply to the extra layers of the uterine lining dries up. The layers start to fall off.

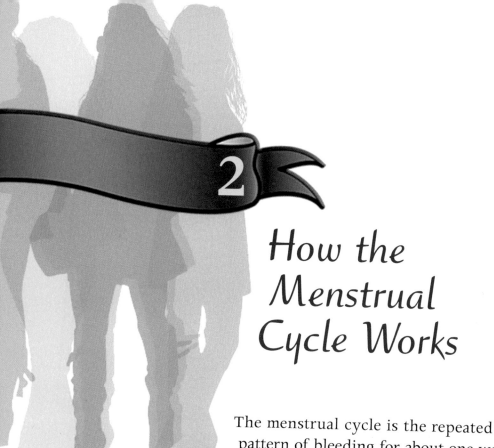

How the Menstrual Cycle Works

The menstrual cycle is the repeated pattern of bleeding for about one week and then not bleeding for a few weeks. We use the term "bleeding" because the discharge looks like blood and contains some blood, but it is mostly tissue from the lining of the uterus. The cycle begins on the first day you start to bleed and lasts until the first day you start to bleed again. For example, if a girl has her first day of bleeding on August 1 and the bleeding for her next period begins August 30, we say she has a thirty-day cycle. The average cycle is twenty-eight days long, but it can be as short as twenty-three days or as long as thirty-five days.

Every girl/woman is unique, and her period may not be like anyone else's in length. It is normal for an individual girl's period and cycle to change and be different from the last one. Some people are very regular, having a period every twenty-eight days

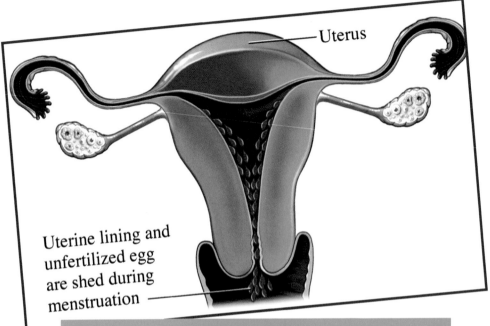

Uterus

Uterine lining and unfertilized egg are shed during menstruation

This illustration shows the female reproductive system during menstruation. The lining of the uterus wall is shed and released.

or every thirty days, for example. Other girls' and women's periods are very different from this. One month a cycle might last twenty-five days, and the next month it might last thirty-two days. Both are normal. When girls first get their periods, the timing is often hard to predict. Sometimes they might skip whole months. This also is normal. It is the way the body settles into its routine pattern. Eventually, most girls have cycles that are fairly regular.

The cycle can be divided into two parts: before the egg is released from the ovary, and after the egg is released. The release of the egg from its follicle is called ovulation.

Before Ovulation

Because so much of what happens during the menstrual cycle is happening inside of the body, we begin counting the cycle from the first easily visible point—the first day a girl begins her menstrual flow, or menses. The first sign of bleeding marks day one of the menstrual cycle. Menses usually lasts from three to five days, sometimes as long as seven days. The flow may be heavy at first, and then taper off. At the beginning of the cycle, the concentration of female hormones in the body is at its lowest point.

When the flow stops, several of the egg follicles in the ovaries begin to develop. The hormone estrogen starts to build up, and the walls of the uterus grow thick and spongy to make a nest for an egg. From about day six to day fourteen, the egg follicles triple in size.

Ovulation

Ovulation occurs when the largest follicle breaks open, releasing a mature egg out of the ovary. It generally takes place fourteen days before the next period begins, no matter how long a girl's cycle is. If someone has a twenty-eight-day cycle, she ovulates on day fifteen. If she has a twenty-four-day cycle, she ovulates on day eleven. A cycle of thirty-five days would mean that she ovulates on day twenty-two. Ovulation can occur twelve to sixteen days before the next period, but for most girls, the number is fourteen. So, the first half of your cycle can be irregular. It can last from nine to twenty-one days. But the second half is always the same, usually fourteen days.

10 Great Questions to Ask Your Doctor

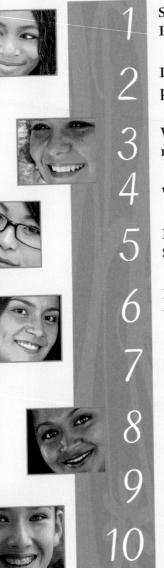

1 Sometimes I see blood clots during my period. Is this OK?

2 I usually spot about two weeks before my period. What does this mean?

3 What can I do to relieve the pain I have during my periods?

4 When will my periods become regular?

5 I am sixteen and haven't had a period yet. Should I just keep waiting?

6 How can I tell if my cramps are normal or if they mean something is wrong?

7 My periods are very heavy. What does that mean?

8 My cramps seem worse every month. Does that mean anything?

9 I have been off birth control for several months. When should my periods start again?

10 I just started taking birth control pills, and I haven't gotten my period. Is this normal?

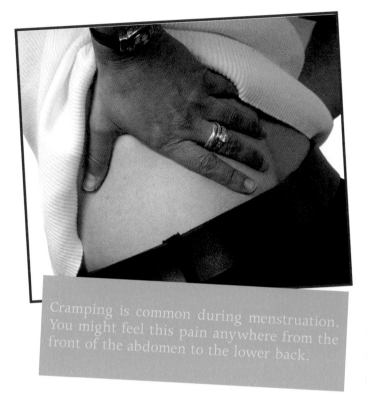

Cramping is common during menstruation. You might feel this pain anywhere from the front of the abdomen to the lower back.

During the time that the body is readying to release an egg and preparing for it to implant in the uterus, other changes occur. Some women and girls may notice changes in the discharge that comes out of the vagina. Around the time that the egg is released, some say they feel a slight pain or cramp in the lower abdomen. Others may have a little spot of blood on their underwear around this time.

The egg lives only twenty-four hours if it is not fertilized. It can be fertilized only after ovulation. But sperm can live longer— at least three days. If a sperm cell is in a female's body when an egg is released, it can fertilize the egg. So, a girl can get pregnant if she has sexual intercourse anytime from three days before ovulation, and maybe more, to one day afterward. Since a girl's cycle can change at any time, if she is sexually active she should use a method of birth control and practice safer sex to avoid unintended pregnancy and sexually transmitted infections (STIs).

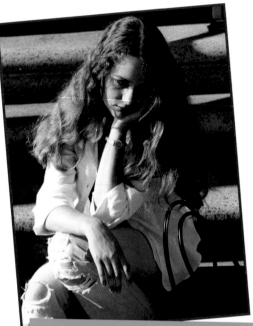

Many girls experience premenstrual syndrome (PMS) due to the changing hormone levels that come with menstruation.

After Ovulation

The part of the cycle after ovulation usually lasts twelve to sixteen days. During this time, the egg makes its way through the fallopian tube to the uterus. The journey takes up to six days. If the egg was not fertilized in the fallopian tube, it will not plant itself in the uterus. But the body does not know if the egg was fertilized, so it gets ready. It assumes that every egg can be a fertilized egg, and numerous hormones are produced. Progesterone is secreted by the ovary and prepares the uterine lining. When the egg and its follicle die, hormone production stops abruptly. Once the body realizes that it does not need the extra materials, it sheds them.

The fairly sharp rise and dip in a girl's hormone level during this time may trigger premenstrual syndrome, or PMS. If a girl has the sad or irritable feelings of PMS, they show up a few days or a week before her period starts. This is the end of the cycle. Sometimes, PMS symptoms continue to bother girls a few days into their periods. The symptoms usually stop when the menses begins or shortly after.

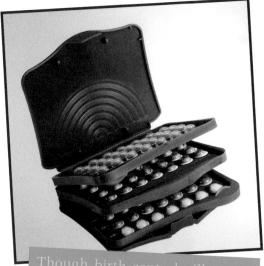

Though birth control pills, such as Seasonale, are designed to prevent pregnancy, one of the side effects may be the regulation of your menstrual cycle.

Birth Control

Though birth control is traditionally used to prevent pregnancy, a side effect that some would consider beneficial is that it can reduce menstruation cycles. The newer forms of birth control on the market that can be used to cut down on menstruation are hormonal and intrauterine. These forms work by altering the body's chemistry.

Though hormonal contraception has been around for years in the form of the Pill, there are new products being developed all the time, including injections of progestin, a synthetic form of the hormone progesterone. Others include a patch that one wears on the buttocks, upper arm, or torso that releases hormones through the skin.

Intrauterine devices (IUDs) are a variant type of hormonal contraception. IUDs are small objects that are inserted into the uterus by a doctor. This form of birth control can work by secreting the hormone progesterone into the body.

There are also nonhormonal intrauterine devices that can help suppress menstruation. The two that are currently on the market are the Copper T 380A (ParaGard) and the levonorgestrel intrauterine system (Mirena). Though nonhormonal IUDs may help to curb menstruation, there are risks that come with their use, including pregnancy complications, pelvic inflammatory disease, and other adverse side effects.

The newest forms of birth control can cut the amount of periods by as much as 70 percent. They are called continuous birth control pills. Though continuous birth control pills may seem like miracle drugs for curbing menstruation, there are risks to be aware of. Some gynecologists predict that they will increase user's estrogen and progesterone exposure over their lifetimes, which may cause unforeseen health complications down the road. However, other gynecologists say that effectively shutting off menstruation is safe.

Since continuous birth control pills are relatively new forms of contraception, only time can tell the true side effects of their use. And, while birth control methods can seem attractive because they shorten or "shut off" menstruation, they should not be used as a means to that end. Though contraceptive medicine is advancing every day, the most effective form of birth control is still, and will always remain, abstinence.

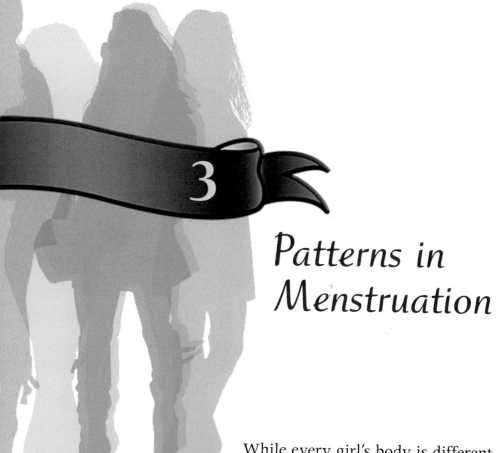

3

Patterns in Menstruation

While every girl's body is different,
menstruation does have predictable
patterns. Most women follow a pattern.
If your menstrual periods seem very different—if you don't get a
period often or have severe cramping, for example—then see a
doctor or another health-care provider.

Getting Your First Period

The female body was made to begin menstruating by about age
sixteen. Typically, a girl will have her first period around age
twelve. The normal range is between ages ten and fourteen. Some
girls start as early as eight, and some as late as sixteen. Beginning
at any age between eight and sixteen is OK. Beginning earlier or
later might be a reason to see a doctor.

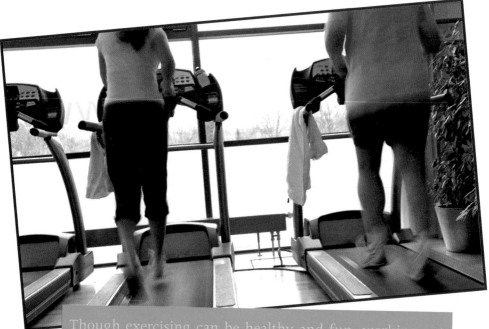

Though exercising can be healthy and fun, working out to the extreme can delay a girl's first period beyond the age of sixteen.

A period before age eight means that a girl has entered puberty, or has begun to mature very early. This is called precocious puberty. Precocious puberty can signal that something unusual is happening in the brain. An injury to the brain can cause the hypothalamus to trigger hormones to begin puberty unusually early. A tumor or infection in the brain can do the same thing. An underactive thyroid gland can also cause a girl to mature early. All of these biological conditions can be treated. Once they are treated, periods stop and normal development resumes.

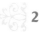

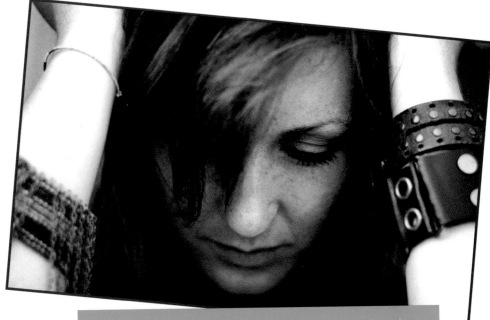

Stress is a part of many people's everyday lives. However, when stress is intense and constant, it can have a negative effect on your menstrual cycle.

Precocious puberty may simply be normal early development for some girls. If your mother or grandmother had her first period early, you probably will, too. If you are of African descent, you usually will start several months or a year before other girls. If you are overweight, you might start early, too.

The reason unusually early puberty is a concern is that it affects how tall a person will be. Bones stop growing after puberty, and early puberty does not give them time to grow very much. Also, developing early sometimes can be hard emotionally and socially.

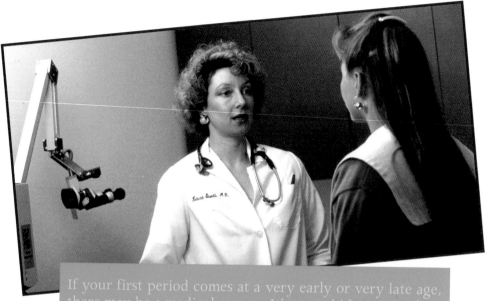

If your first period comes at a very early or very late age, there may be a medical reason. It's a good idea to speak to your doctor to make sure the issue isn't serious.

Doctors will often try to stop this development if it has started too early by prescribing synthetic (man-made) hormones.

On a normal schedule, girls start their periods by age sixteen. As with starting very early, not starting by age sixteen can be caused by a physical disorder. This is usually easy to detect and treat. More often, it happens when a girl is very thin, is exercising to the extreme, or is very stressed. These conditions can be changed.

Whatever the cause, you should see a doctor or other health-care provider if you are sixteen and have not had a period yet. It does not mean something is wrong, but a doctor can make sure everything is working properly. If a girl does not have periods, she will not be able to have children. If she does not start by age sixteen, she can have problems with her bones later in life. The estrogen that is produced during a girl's cycle helps keep calcium in her bones, making them strong. The later a girl begins her periods, the fewer years she has for the estrogen to work. Her bones may not be as strong as they should be and may break more easily when she is older.

Once a girl has her period, and especially if she is sexually active, she should see a gynecologist. A gynecologist is a doctor who specializes in the female reproductive system. Yearly gynecological visits are important to make sure your reproductive system is healthy, to deal with any problems or issues, and to prevent pregnancy or STIs.

How Often Should You Have a Period?

Cycles can be anywhere from twenty-three to thirty-five days. Some cycles are a little shorter or a little longer. When girls first start, their cycles usually tend to be irregular and are often longer than twenty-eight days.

A month might go by without a period. Or you might have two periods very close together. These irregular periods are common, especially when you just start menstruating or when a woman is entering menopause. Usually by the third year, you settle into a regular cycle. Still, your cycle may not always be the same each month. Any big stress, physical or emotional, can delay a period.

The activities you participate in can affect the length of your cycle. These include changes in diet, exercise, and alcohol consumption. Medication can affect your periods. If you are on birth control, that can make a difference. Some birth control pills, injections, and implants can make monthly bleeding stop. Even when you stop taking birth control, periods might not start again for several months.

Some girls always have irregular periods—maybe thirty-two days one month, twenty-one days the next. That is OK. Some girls skip periods fairly often. That is OK, too.

If you've had sex, missing a period could mean that you are pregnant, and you should talk with your doctor. Going three months or more without a period can happen if you are sick, if you suddenly lose a lot of weight, or if you exercise especially hard. It can happen if you have too much stress. But it could also mean your hormones are out of balance because of some physical disorder. One of the most common causes of missed and irregular periods is polycystic ovary syndrome, or PCOS.

Whatever the cause, it is usually treatable. A doctor or other health-care provider can help you understand what is happening to your body and discuss lifestyle and dietary changes with you. You can get well and reduce your stress. You can eat right and exercise more sensibly. A doctor can give you hormones or other medicines that can put you back into a regular rhythm.

How Long and How Heavy Should a Period Be?

For the average girl, a period lasts three to five days. Ten days can be normal. You might have a short period with just a little bleeding for one or two months, and then a longer period with heavier bleeding the next month. When your period is late or you have not had typical periods for a while, your uterus has had longer to build up its lining. When the period does come, your uterus has more than the usual amount of lining to shed. Periods that are further apart are often heavier than periods that are closer together.

You might spot, or bleed just a little, between periods. This is normal. Some people bleed just a little around the time that they ovulate, twelve to sixteen days before their period starts. Heavy bleeding between periods is not common.

You might not know what is light bleeding and what is heavy bleeding. It is usually enough to soak a regular pad or tampon every three to eight hours. If you are soaking a pad or tampon every hour for several hours in a row, your flow is probably too heavy and you should see a doctor.

But you should not worry. Doctors can usually find the cause. It is probably a matter of hormones being out of balance. Whatever it is, it generally can be corrected.

Do not be alarmed if you see clots during your period. These are usually not clots of blood, but pieces of the endometrium. They are very common, especially on the first day of your period.

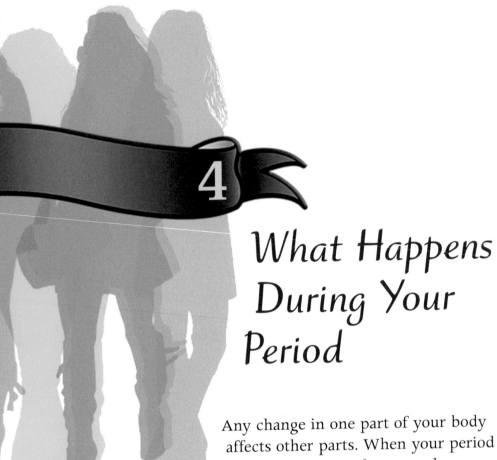

4

What Happens During Your Period

Any change in one part of your body affects other parts. When your period comes every month, many changes take place. These changes can start a chain reaction so that your hair, skin, head, heart, and other organs react. Many physical and emotional experiences come with your period besides bleeding.

Cramps

One of the chemicals in your body makes your uterus contract during your period. This is the same action that pushes a baby out during childbirth. Your uterus needs to contract during your period to force the unneeded uterine lining out. These contractions are what cause cramps. Sometimes the contractions are gentle. Sometimes they are strong.

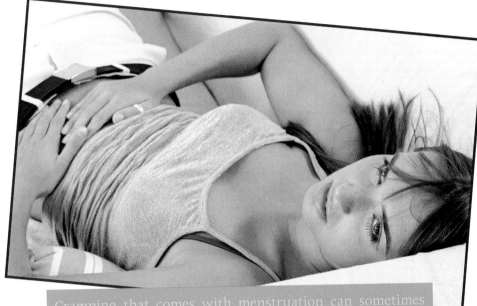

Cramping that comes with menstruation can sometimes feel serious and prevent you from going out. Cramping is normal, though, and lasts only a few days.

If you started having periods early, you are more likely to get cramps. If your period usually lasts a long time and is heavy, you are more prone to cramping.

The kinds of cramps that are most common often start just before or at the very beginning of a period. The pain can be in the lower abdomen, the lower back, the hips, and the thighs. The pain typically is strongest on the first day and often goes away in a day or two. It can hurt a little or a lot, but this does not necessarily signal that something is wrong with your body.

Another kind of pain is more serious and could be a symptom of a condition that needs attention. Some common conditions that can lead to this type of pain are fibroids, which are growths inside the uterus that can be removed; an infection such as pelvic inflammatory disease, which is treatable; or endometriosis or polycystic ovary syndrome (PCOS), both of which can be treated. If any of these conditions cause menstrual pain, the pain goes away when the condition is treated.

Bloating

In addition to cramps, you may feel bloated just before or during your period. If you are bloated, your abdomen feels full and tight. Bloating is usually caused by your body holding on to water. Maybe it needs the extra fluid to build up the uterine lining. Exercising and cutting back on salt and caffeine may help. If not, just wait. The bloating usually goes away when your period is over.

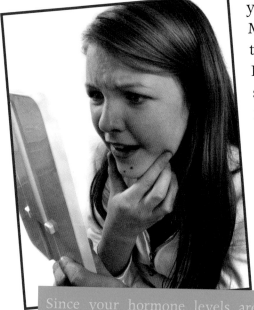

Since your hormone levels are changing during menstruation, you might notice new acne. This is often temporary and leaves with your period.

Pimples

Just before your period, your face might break out. Acne is not caused by menstruation, but it often comes with it. Your hormone level is highest just before your period starts, and those hormones can make acne flare up. Usually, you have fewer pimples as you get older. If acne is a problem for you, talk with your doctor or a dermatologist to see what you can do to reduce outbreaks.

Premenstrual Syndrome

When a condition has a number of different symptoms, and you only need to have one or two symptoms to have the condition, it is called a syndrome. The week or so before your period is your premenstrual time. When a set of symptoms occur during that time, the condition is called premenstrual syndrome, or PMS. You have more hormones in your body the week before your period than when you are actually bleeding. Hormones change when the unfertilized egg decomposes. Your body tries to adjust quickly. As your body adjusts to the changing hormone levels, various symptoms can occur. Common symptoms include headaches, backaches, sore or swollen breasts, diarrhea or constipation. Some people crave certain foods. If you have cramps, bloating, and acne, they could get worse during this time. All these changes can wear you out.

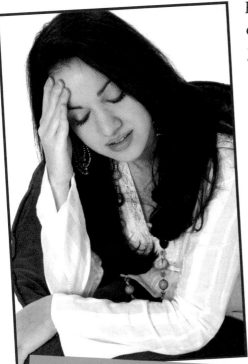

Premenstrual syndrome is one of the more uncomfortable side effects of menstruation. PMS can include physical changes as well as psychological ones.

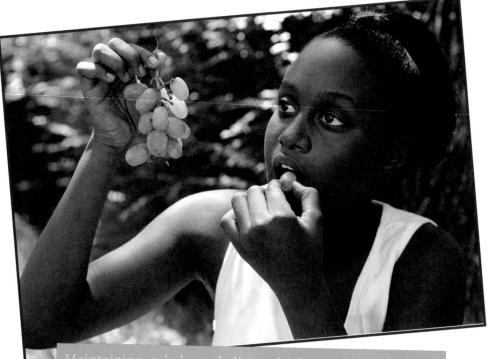

Maintaining a balanced diet, which includes plenty of fruits and vegetables, is a good way to ease the painful effects of PMS and menstruation.

The rapidly changing hormone levels also can make your emotions stronger. Some girls and women feel sad or depressed in the week before their periods, or they may have a hard time concentrating. Many are irritable—they get upset easily. They might snap at others and have a hard time dealing with stress.

Not all these annoyances happen to everyone. You might experience one or two, or you might feel nearly all of them. You might experience none at all.

Premenstrual syndrome generally goes away once the period starts. But females who have PMS usually get it again when the next period comes. What can help you feel better if you have PMS? The same things that reduce any of the discomforts that could come with your period: eating wisely, getting plenty of exercise, and getting enough sleep.

A little discomfort or pain with your period is not uncommon. But if you have so much pain that you cannot go to school or participate in other activities, you probably need to see a doctor. You might have a condition that needs to be treated. Two conditions that cause menstrual pain are endometriosis and polycystic ovary syndrome.

Endometriosis

Endometriosis is a condition in which endometrial tissue grows where it doesn't belong—someplace other than the uterus. It might grow in the ovaries, in the fallopian tubes, or on the outside of the uterus instead of the inside. The tissue develops into growths called implants. As they grow, they put pressure on whatever is around them. That pressure can cause pain. Depending on where they are, the implants can create pain in the abdomen or the lower back. Doctors have not found a way to cure endometriosis, but they can treat it successfully with medication to relieve the symptoms and control the growth of the implants. If the implants are very large and are causing problems, doctors can remove them with surgery. Possibly 20 percent of all women have endometriosis, but only half of them have symptoms that bother them.

Polycystic Ovary Syndrome

Irregular, heavy, and painful periods are sometimes caused by a condition called polycystic ovary syndrome, or PCOS. In PCOS, some of the follicles in the ovaries grow into cysts instead of eggs. Cysts are little sacs filled with fluid. When cysts form, they block the normal release of eggs. This condition can cause other problems such as unwanted hair growth, thinning of hair on the head, and worse acne. In some cases, periods stop altogether.

About 5 to 10 percent of women have PCOS. Doctors can prescribe medicines to regulate the hormones of the body. These medicines usually reduce the formation of cysts so PCOS is no longer a problem. The medication often stops the growth of unwanted hair and the acne.

A Good Sign

Don't think that everything about a period is painful or uncomfortable. Having a period means that you are maturing and healthy. It means that your body is able to have a baby and you may someday be a mother.

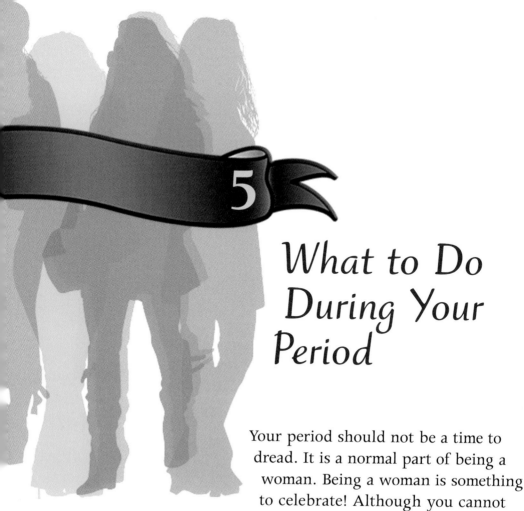

5

What to Do During Your Period

Your period should not be a time to dread. It is a normal part of being a woman. Being a woman is something to celebrate! Although you cannot control when your period will come, you can control some of what the experience will be like.

Using Pads or Tampons

When a girl or woman gets her period, she needs to use something to absorb the blood and other fluids that come out of her body. There are different products to absorb the flow. What you use is entirely up to what you prefer. Pads, also called sanitary napkins, are worn on the outside, in your panties. Tampons are placed inside, in the vagina. Either will work. Some girls don't like using pads because they are bulky, and they leave the wetness and odor of the discharge next to the skin. Others don't like

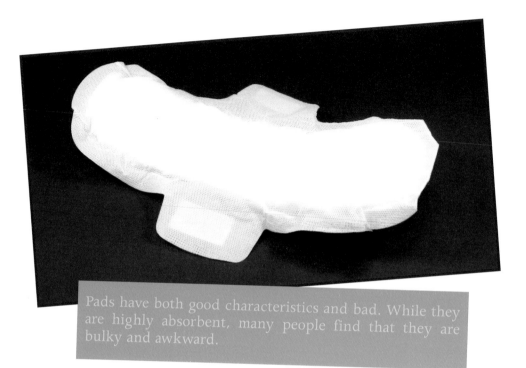

Pads have both good characteristics and bad. While they are highly absorbent, many people find that they are bulky and awkward.

inserting tampons. Many girls who like to swim or play other sports prefer tampons. Use whichever product makes you feel more comfortable.

Both pads and tampons come in different absorbencies, or sizes. It is a good idea to wear the smallest size that will protect your clothes. You can wear maxi pads or super tampons on days your flow is heaviest, and regular pads or tampons on other days. If you are using tampons, you might want to wear a panty liner also, just in case the tampon leaks.

If you are wearing pads, you should change them often. Even on light days when they are not full, change them every four to six hours. This helps eliminate unpleasant odor and helps you feel clean.

Girls who want to use tampons may find them awkward or a little hard to put in at first. Tampons are made of cotton and other absorbent materials. Some are in plastic or cardboard tubes that make them easy to slide into place. With others, you use your fingers to guide them into position. If using a tampon is new for you, just relax. Relaxing is important because you must slip the tampon past the muscles at the bottom of your vagina. If you are tense, those muscles tighten up. Relax and put the tampon in slowly. The muscles will then hold it in place. Make sure you can feel the string on the outside of your body.

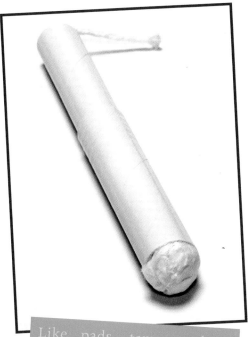

Like pads, tampons have good points and bad. They are less bulky than pads, but some women find them uncomfortable.

Some people may tell you that a virgin cannot use a tampon. Others think that if you use a tampon, you are no longer a virgin. Neither is true. These people are confused about a girl's hymen. The hymen is a thin tissue that covers part of the opening of the vagina. When a girl has sex for the first time, the hymen breaks. It can also break before a girl has sex for the first time. Sometimes putting a tampon in stretches it or breaks it. Breaking the hymen does not change your virginity. Having sexual intercourse is the only thing that affects your virginity.

Toxic Shock Syndrome

Another reason to use the lowest absorbency tampon for your flow is to prevent getting a rare condition, toxic shock syndrome. Toxic shock syndrome, or TSS, is an infection that is caused by bacteria. Doctors are not sure why, but girls and women who use tampons sometimes get it. Those who get it can die from it. TSS begins suddenly and progresses rapidly. The first signs are usually vomiting and a very high fever. A person with TSS often faints or feels dizzy because her blood pressure drops sharply. Her head and muscles usually ache, and she often has diarrhea. Within twenty-four hours, she develops a rash that looks like sunburn, but her skin is cool and moist. She might also have red or bloodshot eyes, and she might seem confused. Because TSS can be deadly, you should go to an emergency room right away if these symptoms appear. The infection can be cured with antibiotics.

Although TSS is rare, you should be careful to lower your risk of getting it. If you use tampons, it is important to change

Toxic shock syndrome, or TSS, usually manifests very quickly. One of the first symptoms of TSS is a high fever.

them frequently. Tampons need to be changed at least every six to eight hours. Do not wear them when you are not on your period. Try wearing mini pads on your lightest days. Always wear the smallest size—the lightest absorbency—that you can for your flow.

Are There Any Activities That Should Be Avoided?

When you are on your period, you are not sick. You are not weak. You can do anything you can do when you are not on your period. You can exercise, play sports, and travel. Some people think they can't go swimming or take a bath. If you wear a tampon, that should not be a problem. There is no health reason not to swim, bathe, or wash your hair during your period.

How to Feel Your Best

The way to feel your best during your period is the same way to feel good all the time: maintain a proper diet, exercise, and rest.

Your body is very busy during this time, and you should give it all the nutrients it needs to stay healthy. Filling your plate with more fresh fruits and vegetables and less fat and sugar is the healthiest way to eat. You might want to cut back on salt as you get close to your period. Salt makes your body retain water, and this can make you feel bloated. In addition, salty foods make you thirsty, so you drink even more water.

Generally, drinking water is good for you as long as you do not have too much salt. If you are bloated, try exercising instead

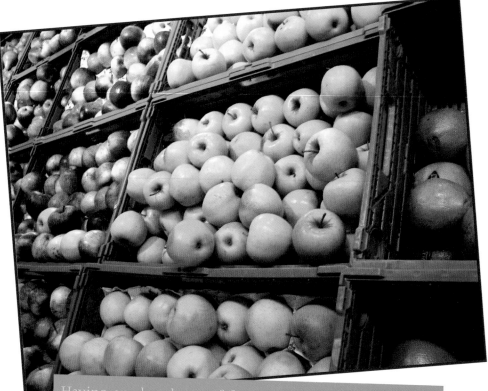

Having an abundance of fruits and vegetables is a great way to curb the effects of PMS and menstruation, since they are loaded with the nutrients you need.

of cutting back on water. If you tend to have PMS, you may want to consider having less caffeine or stopping it altogether. Caffeine is contained in soda, coffee, tea, and chocolate. Caffeine can make you nervous and jumpy. It can make you irritable.

Because menstruating girls lose some blood every month, they need 50 percent more iron than boys. Symptoms of iron deficiency are fatigue, weakness, and headaches. To prevent iron deficiency, you should eat foods high in iron: liver, meat, fish, poultry, eggs, beans, potatoes, spinach, and peas. Some cereals and whole grains have iron in them; so do prunes and raisins. You can buy iron-fortified milk. You should try to like these foods because once you start having periods, you need iron all the time. If you do not get enough iron in your food, you might need to take iron pills. If you are experiencing symptoms of iron deficiency, talk to your doctor.

One of the best things you can do to feel good is exercise. Physical exercise makes all the systems of your body work better. It can relieve cramping and backaches. It can affect hormone production. It can help you sweat out the water that causes bloating. Exercising also makes your body release natural painkillers so you feel good. You can run, dance, cycle, skate, or walk. Don't wait until your period starts. Make exercise a part of your everyday life.

Glossary

cervix The lower section of the uterus that opens into the vagina.

endometrium Membrane that lines the wall of the uterus.

fallopian tube One of two tubes that guide an egg from an ovary to the uterus.

follicle A sac filled with fluid that holds the egg as it matures.

hymen A thin tissue that partly covers the opening of the vagina.

menarche A girl's first menstrual period.

menopause The permanent cessation of a woman's menstrual cycle.

menses The monthly discharge from the uterus.

organ A part of the body that has a special function or purpose.

ovaries Organs in which eggs develop.

ovulation The release of a mature egg from its follicle.

precocious puberty Condition in which the physical changes from a child's body to an adult's body begin earlier than normal.

premenstrual syndrome (PMS) A condition in which a number of physical and emotional changes occur in the week or so before a period.

puberty The period of time, usually between the ages of eight and eighteen, when girls and boys become sexually mature.

ritual A ceremony performed in a certain way.

syndrome A group of symptoms for a particular condition.

uterus The organ in the female body where a fertilized egg grows into a baby.

vagina The canal in the female body that extends from the lower end of the uterus to the outside of the body.

For More Information

American College of Obstetricians and Gynecologists
409 12th Street SW
Washington, DC 20090-6920
(202) 638-5577
Web site: http://www.acog.org

> The American College of Obstetricians and Gynecologists offers fact sheets on health topics.

Center for Young Women's Health
Children's Hospital Boston
333 Longwood Avenue, 5th Floor
Boston, MA 02115
(617) 355-2994
Web site: http://www.youngwomenshealth.org

> The Center for Young Women's Health provides information on the general well-being of girls and young women, including menstruation and gynecological exams.

Endometriosis Association
8585 North 76th Place
Milwaukee, WI 53223
(414) 355-2200
(800) 992-3636
Web site: http://www.endometriosisassn.org

> The Endometriosis Association provides education about the disease.

National Women's Health Information Center
200 Independence Avenue SW
Washington, DC 20201
(800) 944-9662
Web site: http://www.4woman.gov
> This site educates on any topic concerning women's health.

Planned Parenthood Federation of America
434 West 33rd Street
New York, NY 10001
(212) 541-7800
Web site: http://www.plannedparenthood.org
> Planned Parenthood provides comprehensive information on sexual health issues.

Polycystic Ovarian Syndrome Association
P.O. Box 3403
Englewood, CA 80111
Web site: http://www.pcosupport.org
> This association provides information, support, and advocacy for people with PCOS.

Web Sites

Due to the changing nature of Internet links, Rosen Publishing has developed an online list of Web sites related to the subject of this book. This site is updated regularly. Please use this link to access the list:

http://www.rosenlinks.com/gh/mens

For Further Reading

Blume, Judy. *Are You There God? It's Me, Margaret*. New York, NY: Random House Children's Books, 1991.

Fingerson, Laura. *Girls in Power*. Albany, NY: State University of New York Press, 2006.

Fraustino, Lisa Rowe, ed. *Don't Cramp My Style: Stories About "That" Time of the Month*. New York, NY: Simon & Schuster's Children's Publishing, 2004.

Laflamme, Linda. *Rites of Passage: A Celebration of Menarche*. Winchester, MA: Synchronicity Press, 2001.

Madaras, Lynda. *What's Happening to My Body? A Growing-Up Guide for Parents and Daughters*. New York, NY: Newmarket Press, 2000.

Bibliography

Christensen, Barbara Lauritsen, and Elaine Oden Kockrow, eds. *Foundations of Nursing,* Third Edition. New York, NY: Mosby, 1999.

Early, P. J. "Most Often, 'Early Puberty' Still Normal." HealthLink. Retrieved March 24, 2006. (http://healthlink.mcw.edu/article/1031002256.html).

Goseyun, Anna Early. "Case Study: Sunrise Ceremonial." Historical Society of Pennsylvania. Retrieved March 1, 2006 (http://www2.hsp.org/exhibits/Balch%20exhibits/rites/apache.html).

Reaves, Malik Stan. "Alternative Rite to Female Circumcision in Kenya." African News Service. November 19, 1997. Retrieved March 1, 2006 (http://fr.allafrica.com/stories/200101080370.htm).

"Rites of Passage." Fact Monster. Retrieved March 15, 2006 (http://www.factmonster.com/ipka/A0906923.html).

Simon, Harvey. "Menstruation." Well Connected Reports. 2002. Retrieved April 1, 2006 (http://umm.edu/patiented/articles).

Thomas, Clayton L., ed. *Taber's Cyclopedic Medical Dictionary.* Philadelphia, PA: F. A. Davis, 1997.

Index

Photo Credits

Designer: Evelyn Horovicz; **Editor:** Nicholas Croce
Photo Research: Amy Feinberg